Is It Tomorrow Yet?

Paradoxes of the Pandemic

IVAN KRASTEV

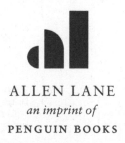

ALLEN LANE
an imprint of
PENGUIN BOOKS

ALLEN LANE

UK | USA | Canada | Ireland | Australia
India | New Zealand | South Africa

Allen Lane is part of the Penguin Random House group of companies
whose addresses can be found at global.penguinrandomhouse.com

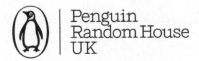

Penguin
Random House
UK

First published 2020
001

Copyright © Ivan Krastev, 2020

The moral right of the author has been asserted

Set in 12.5/14.75 pt Garamond MT Std
Typeset by Jouve (UK), Milton Keynes
Printed and bound in Great Britain by Clays Ltd, Elcograf S.p.A.

A CIP catalogue record for this book is available from the British Library

ISBN: 978-0-241-48345-9

www.greenpenguin.co.uk

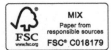

MIX
Paper from
responsible sources
FSC® C018179

Penguin Random House is committed to a
sustainable future for our business, our readers
and our planet. This book is made from Forest
Stewardship Council® certified paper.

To Boris, Lilli and Svetoslav Bojilov, and my family – Yoto, Niya and Dessy – with whom we spent several unforgettable weeks, living through a quarantine together and reflecting upon the coronavirus crisis that was unfolding before our eyes.

Man is the only known time machine.

Georgi Gospodinov, *Time Shelter*

Contents

1   The Return of the Unresolved   1

2   Stay-at-Home Nationalism   19

3   Democracy as a Dictatorship of
    Comparisons   35

4   Are You Here?   65

    Notes   73

    Acknowledgements   79

1. The Return of the Unresolved

Epidemics infect society with fear. Though they can bring out the best in people, they can also bring out the worst in governments. In José Saramago's novel *Blindness*,[1] a man suddenly loses his sight, as does the doctor who examines him and a thief who steals his car, and in no time life descends into chaos. Fearful of the spread of the 'white sickness', the government takes draconian measures to halt the contagion. All those who are already blind and those who have had contact with them are rounded up and taken to a former mental asylum at the edge of the city. Any attempt to leave the hospital is met with lethal force from patrolling soldiers, petrified that they will also lose their sight. The asylum becomes more of a concentration camp than a hospital.

In the novel's final pages, the epidemic abates as suddenly as it began, leaving people to wonder why they became blind. 'I don't think we did go blind, I think we are blind, blind but seeing,' concludes one of the characters. 'Blind people who can see, but do not see.'[2] Saramago doesn't believe that epidemics transform society; in his view, they help us to see the truth about our societies. If he is right, the COVID-19 pandemic should have opened our eyes to the world we have been living in. It should have helped us to make sense of it.

'The first thing that plague brought to our town was exile,' notes the narrator in Camus's *The Plague*,[3] and these days we have a decent sense of what he meant. A society in quarantine is literally a 'closed society'. Many people cease working, they stop meeting their friends and relatives, they quit driving their cars, and they put their lives on hold.

The one thing that we absolutely cannot stop doing is talking about the virus that threatens to change our world for ever. We are imprisoned in our homes, haunted by fear, boredom and paranoia. Benevolent (and not-so-benevolent) governments closely follow where we go and whom we meet, determined to protect us from both our own recklessness and the recklessness of our fellow citizens. Unsanctioned walks in the park may elicit fines or even jail time, and contact with other people has become a threat to our very existence. The unsolicited touching of others is tantamount to betrayal. As Camus observed, the plague erased the 'uniqueness of each man's life' as it heightened our awareness of our vulnerability and powerlessness to plan for the future.[4] After an epidemic, all those still living are survivors.

But for how long will the memory of this unprecedented social experiment last? Could it be that in just a few years we'll remember it as a kind of mass hallucination caused by 'a shortage of space made up for by a surplus of time', as the poet Joseph Brodsky once described a prisoner's existence?

The COVID-19 pandemic has turned out to be a classic 'grey swan event' – highly probable and capable of turning our world upside down, but nonetheless a huge shock when it arrives. In 2004, the US National Intelligence Council predicted that 'it is only a matter of time before a new pandemic appears, such as the 1918–19 influenza virus that killed an estimated 20 million worldwide',* and that such an occurrence could 'put a halt to global travel and trade during an extended period, prompting governments to expend enormous resources on overwhelmed health sectors'. In a 2015 TED Talk, Bill Gates predicted not only a global epidemic of a highly infectious virus, but also warned us that we were unprepared to respond to it. Hollywood also presented us with its own blockbuster 'warnings'. But it's no accident that there are no grey swans in *Swan Lake*; 'grey swans' are an example of something predictable yet unthinkable.

Although great epidemics are, in fact, not such rare occurrences, for some reason their arrival always surprises us. They reset our world in a similar way to wars and revolutions, yet these other things stamp

---

* The estimates of the number of victims of Spanish flu vary significantly.

themselves on our collective memory in a manner that epidemics somehow do not. In her marvellous book *Pale Rider*, the science writer Laura Spinney shows that the Spanish flu was the most tragic event in the twentieth century but is now mostly forgotten. A century ago, the pandemic infected a third of the world's population, a staggering 500 million people. Between the first recorded case on 4 March 1918 and the last in March 1920, the pandemic wiped out between 50 and 100 million people. In terms of loss of life from a single event, it surpassed both the First World War (17 million dead) and the Second World War (60 million dead) and may have killed as many people as both wars put together. Yet, as Spinney notes, 'When asked what was the biggest disaster of the twentieth century, almost nobody answers the Spanish flu.'[5] More surprisingly, even historians seem to have forgotten the epidemic. In 2017, WorldCat, the world's largest library catalogue, listed roughly 80,000 books on the First World War (in more than forty languages) but barely 400 on the Spanish flu (in five languages). How can it be that an epidemic that killed at least five times more people than died in the First World War has resulted in 200 times fewer books? Why do we remember wars and revolutions but forget pandemics, even though the latter change our economies, politics, societies and urban architecture just as fundamentally?

Spinney believes that one key reason is that it's

easier to count those killed by bullets than those who die from a virus, and the present controversy regarding the mortality rate of COVID-19 seems to suggest that she is right. The other, more fundamental, reason is that it's difficult to turn a pandemic into a good story. It is impossible to retell it as a clash of good and evil. It lacks a plot and a moral. In 2015, the psychologists Henry Roediger and Magdalena Abel suggested that people tend to remember only 'a small number of salient events' from any situation, namely those 'referring to beginning, turning and end points'.[6] It's very hard to tell the story of the Spanish flu (or of any other great epidemic, for that matter) with this narrative structure; epidemics are like Netflix series, where the end of one season is merely a hiatus before the next one. The relationship between the epidemic and war resembles the relationship between some modernist literature and the classical novel. The strangeness of the pandemic experience is that everything changes but nothing happens. We are asked to save humanity by staying home and washing our hands. As in a modernist novel, all the action is in the mind of the narrator.

Our inability, or perhaps our unwillingness, to remember epidemics might also have something to do with our general aversion to random death and suffering. 'Dying is an art, like everything else,' writes Sylvia Plath. But is this also true in the plague times? 'The global fight against COVID-19 is not a life-or-death battle,' says the scientist Carlo Rovelli, because 'Death always wins in the end; we are mortal. What is going on is the great effort of all of us to give each other some more time – for this short life, despite suffering and hardships, seems more beautiful to us than ever.'[7] The meaninglessness of arbitrary pain is hard to bear; the victims of the current epidemic suffer not only a tragic demise because they're unable to breathe, but also because nobody can really explain the meaning of their death. War comes with the promise of heroic victory. In the patriotic narrative, soldiers don't just die – they sacrifice their lives for others. The story of wars is one of ordinary people demonstrating extraordinary courage by sacrificing their lives in order to save others. William James called war 'the gory nurse that trained societies in cohesiveness'. In a plague, however, there's nothing heroic. So, unsurprisingly, when societies try to remember a plague, they memorialize it as a kind of war. There is a type of monument in the history of art called a 'plague column', such as the one on the Graben in Vienna. Tellingly, they are often described as 'monuments to celebrate victory over the plague'.

But COVID-19 not only brings meaningless death; it also brings undignified death. In all testimonies of plague years, it is the fact that people die without a proper funeral that compounds the tragedy for contemporary chroniclers. It's no different this time. The fear of infection has made many family members reluctant to attend the funerals of their relatives, and on many occasions there are no funerals at all or there are Zoom funerals.

Deja Vu *All Over Again*

We have precious few clues as to when the COVID-19 pandemic will end, and nor do we know *how* it will end. If we're using the Spanish flu as our yardstick, the pandemic has not even arrived yet. The great die-offs and social shocks still lie in the future.

At present, we're able only to speculate about its long-term political and economic impact. Historians are clear that 'a true epidemic is an event, not a trend': as the medical historian Charles Rosenberg puts it, 'Epidemics start at a moment in time, proceed on a stage limited in space and duration, follow a plot line of increasing revelatory tension, move to a crisis of individual and collective character, then drift toward closure.'[8] The truth of the matter is that COVID-19 *will* change our world in profound ways, regardless of whether or not we remember the days of pandemic. The world will be transformed not because our societies want change or because there's a consensus for the direction of change – but because we cannot go back.

In the twenty-first century, we have already heard that our world was going to be altered for ever three times: after 9/11, after the Great Recession of 2008–9, and in Europe following the refugee crisis of 2015. The claim that the world 'will never be the same again' is in one sense simply a prediction that many things are about to change, although we know full well that things change all the time. It also means something much more concrete: the end of the liberal world order that was born out of the collapse of the Berlin Wall, a world characterized by the global spread of democracy and capitalism and shaped by the power and will of America and its European allies. During all previous crises, pundits claimed that the liberal order was dead. At times it seemed to be in intensive care, but it always retained the capacity to recover. Why should this time be any different?

Is it not true that, of all the crises threatening humanity, COVID-19 may be the most globalization-friendly in terms of the evidence it provides for the importance of international cooperation? Unlike wars, pandemics don't pit nations against each other. Unlike great migrations, they don't cause violent nationalism. And, unlike earthquakes or tsunamis, pandemics are global. A pandemic is a crisis that allows humanity to experience its interdependence and its togetherness. It places humanity's hope in science and rationality. Is it the pandemic itself, or is it the failure of the world's political leaders to mobilize a collective response to the crisis, that makes us pessimistic about the future?

In mid-March 2020, profoundly disturbed by the spread of the pandemic and safely ensconced in a friend's house in the Bulgarian countryside, I became vexed by the question of how COVID-19 would change the world. I saw the post-coronavirus world as one in which certain trends and conflicts that were present before the virus arrived would be intensified; in this sense, I see the virus as an amplifier rather than a disrupter. I argued that COVID-19 would end a disruptive decade marked by the unravelling of globalization and cause profound changes to our politics, economies and ways of life. I anticipated the return of the state, backed by a restored trust in expertise and scientific knowledge. I also sensed the rise of nationalism and the blurring of the borders between democracy and big-data authoritarianism. Like many others, I expected the decline of America's global dominance (though I didn't necessarily predict America's current breakdown). It was my understanding that the coronavirus will challenge some of the basic assumptions upon which the European Union was founded, which could be a prelude to a major transformation of the European project. If things go wrong, COVID-19 could trigger the disintegration of the European Union; if they go right, it could consolidate the Union.[9]

How did my early conjectures fare? I began by articulating seven early lessons; one quarantine later, these lessons have been reconceptualized into seven paradoxes.

1. COVID-19 exposes the dark side of globalization – but also acts as an agent of globalization. The virus is most vicious in places that are, according to historian Frank Snowden, 'densely populated and linked by rapid air travel, by movements of tourists, of refugees, all kinds of businesspeople, all kinds of interlocking networks'. At the same time, it has synchronized the world and brought us together in a way no previous crisis could. For some time we have lived in a common world.

2. The pandemic has accelerated the trend towards de-globalization that was triggered by the Great Recession of 2008–9, while at the same time exposing the limits of re-nationalization. In a post-COVID-19 world, Gideon Rachman surmises that 'It is hard to believe that large developed countries will continue to accept a situation in which they have to import most of their vital medical supplies.' If the high point of globalization in the 1990s was represented (at least in the public imagination) by the efficiencies of just-in-time global supply chains, then today the public is seduced by the image of a

strong state that can stockpile all the
resources society needs in a crisis.

3. Fear of the virus in the early stages of the
   pandemic inspired a state of national unity
   that many societies have not experienced in
   years, but in the longer term it will deepen
   existing social and political divides. The
   pandemic will not only intensify the political,
   economic and social divisions that were
   once manifest throughout all societies – it
   will also establish the pandemic as a line in
   the sand. And the more the fear of COVID-19
   recedes, the less we will acknowledge that
   the threat was ever real. The paradox is that
   the countries that were either most effective
   in containing the virus or were most lucky
   to be less affected by it will be the places
   where public opinion will be most eager to
   criticize the government for its lockdown
   policies.

4. COVID-19 has put democracy on hold, at
   least in Europe, with many countries enacting
   a state of emergency; but by doing so, it
   limited people's desire for more authoritarian
   government. One consequence of civil rights
   and liberties being frozen will be a rejection
   rather than an embrace of authoritarianism.
   In the early stages of the crisis, people
   willingly granted extraordinary powers to

their governments, but they will become increasingly uncharitable as economic concerns begin to supplant public health ones. This is the changing nature of the COVID-19 calamity: a health disaster that turns into an economic one makes the political consequences of the crisis incredibly difficult to predict.

5. The pandemic initially restored trust in expertise and science, while at the same time it produced some of the most shocking conspiracy theories. The outcome is that, while governments and experts view the arrival of a vaccine as the only real end of the crisis, only 49 per cent of Americans declare readiness to vaccinate themselves.

6. While the EU was notably absent in the early stages of the crisis, the pandemic has become more critical for the future of the Union than anything in its history. The EU is not just risking territorial disintegration, as in Brexit, but a slide into irrelevance. But at the same time, it is COVID-19 that has brought Europe's 'Hamiltonian moment' and has pushed the process of European integration.

7. While the EU views itself as the 'last man standing' in defence of openness and interdependence, it could be the pressure of

de-globalization rather than commitment to liberal values that pushes Europeans to adopt more common policies and even to hand over some emergency powers to Brussels.

Contemplating the possible changes that COVID-19 might inspire, I was reminded of a line from Stephen Leacock's *Nonsense Novels*: 'Lord Ronald said nothing; he flung himself from the room, flung himself upon his horse, and rode madly off in all directions.'

Be Realistic: Demand the Impossible

There are moments when our certainties break down and our collective notion of what is possible changes dramatically. People begin to ignore the present and instead start thinking about the future, whether that's what they hope for or what they fear.

It took a virus to turn the world on its head: as I mentioned, the EU was temporarily suspended and citizens took shelter in the security of the nation state: democracy was put on hold, emergency legislation was introduced in most European countries, parliamentarians have been sent home, demonstrations outlawed and elections postponed, and opposition parties have lost political relevance. It was also a world in which capitalism was temporarily suspended, with unemployment skyrocketing and the global economy undergoing a crisis far more devastating than the Great Recession of 2008–9. Indeed, governmental 'interference' in economic markets is more prevalent today than at any time since 1989, and temporary nationalization has become the new normal.

Today we are able to imagine anything because we are being besieged by something that was considered unimaginable. We are suddenly able to imagine that the United States could achieve universal healthcare, that China could overtake the United States as the world's most significant power, that Russian president Vladimir Putin could lose power or that the European Union could either collapse or become a 'United States of Europe'. As planes are grounded and the big polluting corporations have closed their production lines, climate activists have started to believe that their dreams of a low-carbon world are achievable. And when the borders between the EU member states are closed, right-wing populists begin to feel that they might never be reopened.

As the filmmaker and activist Astra Taylor has put it,

[the] response to the coronavirus pandemic has revealed a simple truth: so many policies that our elected officials have long told us were impossible and impractical were eminently possible and prac-

tical all along . . . Now, we know that the 'rules' we
have lived under were unnecessary . . . This is an
unprecedented opportunity to not just hit the pause
button and temporally ease the pain, but to permanently change the rules.[10]

It's an opportunity, but it's a grave risk, too.

Panic and Triviality

Politics is not like art. In art, 'habitual perception kills,'
argued Viktor Shklovsky, the Russian twentieth-
century literary theorist. 'It devours works, clothes,
furniture, one's wife and the fear of war.' Shklovsky
believed that a work of art possessed the ability to
make the familiar look unfamiliar, forcing us to see
the usual through fresh eyes.[11] Politics works the
other way around: it makes us regard the unfamiliar
as familiar. Art excites the public about the 'normal',
while politics trivializes the exceptional. It is no
longer a secret that 'men are ruled by . . . the weakness of their imagination'.[12]

In this context, COVID-19 shakes politicians out
of their usual modus operandi. In order to mobilize
public opinion, they are forced to insist that this crisis is unprecedented even in countries in which the
numbers of infected and dead are currently very low
(like my own country, Bulgaria). At the same time, in

order to persuade people that they are capable of resolving the crisis in all its multiple dimensions, European governments are tending to portray COVID-19 as the simultaneous second coming of the three previous crises that shattered the old continent in the last decade – terrorism, the financial crisis and the refugee crisis.

By declaring that the virus is the 'invisible enemy' and by applying the sorts of surveillance technology previously used for detecting terrorists to track the spread of the disease, governments have made people feel that coronavirus is a new sort of terrorism. In a similar way, the closing of the borders between EU member states in response to the pandemic recalls the refugee crisis of 2015 and the fear of the spread of ethnic nationalism.

Finally, the debate in Europe about 'coronabonds' suggests that what we're witnessing today is a financial crisis similar to the Great Recession. But while the economic consequences of the COVID-19 crisis in many ways resemble the Great Recession, economists agree that the current economic crisis is not just deeper than but fundamentally different from the previous one. The pandemic has disrupted global supply chains and caused a simultaneous crisis of demand and supply that will lead to high unemployment. As the economic historian Adam Tooze has pointed out, 'There has never been a crash landing like this before. There is something new under the

sun. And it is horrifying. '[13] In a similar way, the re-
actions of citizens to governments' restrictions of their
rights differ significantly in the context of the corona
crisis in comparison with the 'war on terror'. And the
nationalism triggered by COVID-19 is profoundly
different from the ethnic nationalism triggered by
the refugee crisis. But driven by the instinct to deal
with uncertainty by making the unfamiliar look
familiar, politicians committed a grave mistake,
because COVID-19 went much deeper under the
public's skin than any of the previous crises.

This slim book is not a prediction about the shape
of the world post-COVID-19, nor is it a manifesto for
the future. What I want to do is analyse the COVID-
19 calamity as a new phenomenon, fundamentally
different from the previous three crises. And this is
mainly a book about Europe, while making it clear
that the pandemic is not a European crisis. COVID-
19 is a *global* crisis in the most literal sense of the word.
It is everybody's crisis. The United Nations World
Food Programme has warned that the number of
people facing acute food insecurity and hunger could
double by the end of 2020, to 265 million people. We
may witness a wave of political and military conflicts.
We should expect new waves of migration. And yet I
think that it is in Europe that COVID-19 will have its
most radical political impact, because the pandemic
challenges the foundations on which the European
project is built: namely that interdependency is the

most reliable source of security and prosperity. It is for this reason that I believe that the European Union is not going to be the same after this crisis. It could disintegrate, it could be transformed into a twenty-first-century copy of the medieval Holy Roman Empire, a union in name only, or it could achieve its long-dreamt-of strategic autonomy.

2. Stay-at-Home Nationalism

In early April 2020, the journalist Chiara Pagano noted drily that, 'Italy is now more closed than Matteo Salvini ever dreamed it would be.'[1] She had a point. Over the course of a single week, COVID-19 closed more European borders than the continent's refugee crisis in 2015 ever managed. In the month of March, air travel in Europe plummeted a staggering 97 per cent compared to the previous month. Many liberals consider this decline in travel a tragedy of real consequence; the coronavirus has infected the continent with an incurable nationalism that is now threatening the very survival of the European Union, and its malevolent spread confirms the mystique of borders.

The refugee crisis in 2015 fundamentally destabilized the European project, fuelling the division between those who advocated freedom of movement and those who pressed for closing state borders and widening the gap between Eastern and Western Europe. Over the course of the crisis, a majority of Europeans lost confidence in the assumed virtue of globalization.

The tourist and the refugee have become the

symbols of the contrasting faces of globalization. Tourists exemplify 'good globalization', and are welcomed with open arms. These benevolent foreigners come, spend, admire and leave, making us feel connected to a larger world without imposing its problems on us. By contrast, refugees represent the threatening nature of globalization.[2] They come weighed down by the misery of the wider world. They are among us, but they are not of us. They make claims on our resources and force us to confront the limits of our solidarity.

Attracting tourists and rejecting migrants is a greatly simplified version of Europe's desired world order. However, during the COVID-19 pandemic, refugees are still crowding at the gates of Europe, while tourists have vanished. The long-term consequences of the crisis will probably be that the economic freefall caused by the pandemic will increase pressure on Europe's borders.

The Global South will probably be the major victim of the economic slowdown. The price of natural resources is in free fall, and the value of remittances is expected to fall by around 20 per cent, compared with 5 per cent during the global financial crisis of 2008, and the withdrawal of foreign investment will impel people to seek opportunities outside their own countries. At the same time, the prospect of tourists returning to Europe in the near future is bleak. Europeans will encounter more migrants on their borders at a time when the closing of borders is not an expression of a lack of solidarity but rather the geopolitical version of 'social distancing'. This could result in the victory of ethnic nationalism and nativist populism in European politics.

The European Union emerged from the violent crucible of European nationalism, which explains why many pro-Europeans have a strong aversion to any idea that carries even a slight whiff of nationalism. The fears of liberals that the coronavirus pandemic will cause an outbreak of flag-waving are not hard to understand, especially if we bear in mind that xenophobia has historically accompanied epidemics. And, just like clockwork, such outbursts have been common in the current pandemic. In Italy, the immigrant Chinese population was blamed for what became labelled as the 'Wuhan virus'. However, in historical terms, the early stages of this pandemic may be remembered less for the rise of xenophobia than for the absence of any eruption of the politics of ethnic hate. It is not the rise of nationalism but rather the exposure of the limits of economic nationalism this crisis will be remembered for.

Where is Home?

Most of us have never experienced a war or a military coup first-hand, but we all instinctively know that a citizen's impulse at a moment of profound danger is to embrace the closing of national borders. By taking such action, politicians declare their readiness to take responsibility for what is happening in their own states. And just as people seek shelter in their country, they also look for shelter in their native language. Psychologists have shown that people often revert to speaking in their mother tongue in moments of great imperilment. During my own childhood in Bulgaria, I learned a valuable lesson from watching scores of Soviet films about the Second World War. One of the most dangerous moments for Soviet female spies in Hitler's Reich was childbirth, because they would involuntarily cry out in their native Russian.

The message urging people to 'stay at home' has encouraged them to define their home not just in pragmatic terms – the best place to live and work – but also in a metaphysical sense. Home is the place where we most want to be during a time of grave danger. It took me by surprise that, as it became clear that the coronavirus was a pandemic and we were probably facing a prolonged period of social distancing, my family decided to go back to Bulgaria before the lockdown. In many respects this was not a rational decision. We have lived and worked in Vienna for a decade and love the city; the Austrian public health system is far more reliable than the system in Bulgaria, and we could depend on our friends in the city. Yet what brought us back to Bulgaria was the understanding that we should 'stay at home', and Bulgaria *is* home for us. In a time of crisis, we wanted to be closer to the people and places that we have known all our lives. We weren't alone: 200,000 Bulgarians living abroad did the same thing.

Closing borders is not just historical instinct; it's also the most traditional way of fighting epidemics. It's the way in which states practise social distancing. In 1710, the Holy Roman Emperor Joseph I decided to block the spread of disease from the Balkans by creating a *cordon sanitaire* along the Habsburg Empire's southern frontier with the Ottoman Empire. His actions were largely successful, though they failed to save his own life; he died of smallpox in 1711. Nonetheless, the empire's restrictions on movement lasted until the mid-nineteenth century. And the authorities strictly imposed it.

One English observer noted: 'If you dare to break the laws of the quarantine, you will be tried with military haste; the court will scream out a sentence to you from a tribunal some fifty yards off . . . and after that you will find yourself carefully shot and carelessly buried.'[3]

In the days of Europe's refugee crisis in 2015, nationalism came in the guise of a culture war. It was 'us' versus 'them', and the tone was aggressive. Nationalists made anxious claims about the destruction of their national cultures by foreigners. Bulgarians living outside Bulgaria were part of the 'we', while minorities living in the country – many of whom had been there for centuries – were treated as foreigners. COVID-19 has replaced this cultural nationalism with a public health-oriented nationalism combined with an inverted xenophobia that is territorial in its nature and more inclusive. The foreigner is no longer the person who was not born here, but the one who is not here now – it's your residence rather than your passport that matters. Portugal is a great example of this turn. On the day the Portuguese government locked down the country, it declared that all foreigners with pending applications would be treated as permanent residents until at least 1 July. During the refugee crisis, public debates in many countries were stirred by imagining those who have not yet come – but could. In this crisis, the only migrants who matter are those already in the country.[4]

As I argued in *After Europe*, the anti-foreigner hysteria that marked the response to the 2015 refugee crisis in Central Europe was rooted in the trauma of emigration: many young East Europeans moved to live and work in the West after the end of the Cold War. Fears of depopulation and a sense of abandonment are apparent in our current crisis, too. The coronavirus has made the exodus of medical professionals from Central and Eastern Europe painfully evident. As a result, almost half of the doctors and nurses in countries such as Bulgaria are over fifty years old. But while Bulgarians, Romanians and Poles used to dream that their co-nationals would return during the refugee crisis, in the dark days of COVID-19 the hope is that they will come back only once the virus has been conquered. Co-nationals returning from corona-infected areas have been as unwelcome as any foreigner, and governments have made it clear that during the pandemic they will take responsibility only for those citizens who have decided to stay within the walls of the city. Bulgarian citizens who, for whatever reason, have decided to stay outside the country are no longer regarded as being their government's responsibility.

In this sense, the early stages of the coronavirus crisis were marked not by criticism of foreigners by 'natives', but by the anger of those living in the countryside at the invasion of the 'second-homers'. The media regularly reported on affluent city dwellers decamping from the epicentres of the crisis to their second homes, where proximity to the coast or the mountains would lessen the discomfort of confinement – and a decent internet link would permit remote work. Yet their arrival enraged local residents, because of a fear that they would spread the virus to areas with fewer hospitals that could not withstand a surge of sick, older locals with limited incomes. France, with its 3.4 million second homes, is a vivid illustration of a place where the decision of the affluent middle class to escape the country's major urban centres has been viewed as one more indication of the arrogance and selfishness of those with money.

The uncomfortable irony is that second homes in Europe are themselves a legacy of plague. After the first few outbreaks of the fourteenth-century Black Death, many inhabitants of cities in Renaissance Italy began to invest in country estates, partly to secure reliable food supplies in times of crisis. They spent increasing amounts of time in the countryside, especially during the summer months when the plague was at its worst, and villa life became popular for wealthier families. In the current pandemic, second homes have once again become safe havens, and this time the locals aren't at all pleased.

The Return of Big Government

The rise of a pandemic-triggered nationalism has contributed significantly to the return to prominence of the nation state. After the collapse of Lehman Brothers and Bear Stearns in 2008, many observers believed that mistrust in the financial markets would inexorably lead to greater faith in government. The concept was not a new one. In 1929, following the onset of the Great Depression, people demanded strong intervention from governments to offset the failings of the market. In the 1970s it was the other way around: people were disappointed with government intervention, so the market returned to strength before arriving with a vengeance in the following decade, with Reagan and Thatcher leading the crusade. The paradox of the Great Recession of 2008–9 is that mistrust in the market did not lead to pressure for greater government intervention. Despite the call from Occupy activists all over the world that politics and society be reimagined, the state was not tasked with this responsibility.

Europe's ideological experience of economic recession resonates with a story in Giovanni Boccaccio's great set of tales, *The Decameron*. Giannotto di Civignì makes it his mission to convert his friend Abraham, a Parisian Jew, to Christianity in order to save his soul. One day Abraham departs for Rome, telling Giannotto that he shall only decide whether he wants to convert once he has seen the leaders of the church. Aware of the corruption of the Catholic clergy, Giannotto loses hope that Abraham will make the move. Yet upon his return Abraham does convert, concluding that if Christianity can still thrive when its hierarchy is corrupt, it is probably the true word of God.

We might recognize that something similar has happened to neoliberalism in the wake of the global financial crisis of 2008–9. Many Europeans used to think that, if neoliberalism could somehow survive unscathed after the economic devastation it helped cause, it might as well be *the* true religion; but, just a decade on, COVID-19 has impelled people to re-assess the role of government in their lives. As a result of the pandemic, people rely on the government to organize their collective public health and depend on governmental institutions to save economies that are in freefall. In an interesting twist, the effectiveness of governments is now measured by their capacity to change people's everyday behaviour; in the context of this crisis, inaction is the most visible action. People have demonstrated a readiness to tolerate significant restrictions to their rights, but they do not tolerate governments that are not prepared to take action.

Two aspects of the COVID-19 crisis have gone unnoticed and made observers believe that the virus has infected societies with ethnic national-ism. The first is that, while the politics of social distancing gives extraordinary powers to national governments, it also strengthens the presence of local governments and regional identities. Second, the closing of European borders may expose the limits of nationalism. At a time when economic anxiety dominates public debate, Europeans may realize that, unlike in the nineteenth century, nationalism is economically unsustainable. The United States and China can entertain the illusion of self-sufficiency when it comes to their respective economies, and the European Union could also benefit from careful 'de-globalization', but small European nation states won't stand a chance. Europeans will soon realize that the only protection available to them is the sort of protectionism provided by their association with the rest of the continent. Sweden is the classical example of the limits of any economic nationalism. While the government in Stockholm, contrary to its neighbours, decided not to lockdown the country, hoping to limit the economic costs of the quarantine, the outcome of their action will be the opposite of the expected – Sweden's economic decline in 2020 will be worse than that of some of the EU members who totally closed their economies for weeks.

At Home, in Different Rooms

Looked at from afar, coronavirus seems fundamentally egalitarian. Unlike diseases such as cholera, it doesn't target crowded urban tenements populated by poor people and served by contaminated water supplies. Rather, it doesn't discriminate, attacking rich and poor alike. A closer look forces us to change this perception. The virus has struck societies that are torn apart by different kinds of inequality, and early data from the US powerfully demonstrates that income and race play an important role when it comes to who will die. As Stephen Holmes argues, the pandemic highlights the unequal 'distribution of danger' in society – downward mobility into the grave – rather than merely the unequal distribution of resources and chances for upward mobility.[5]

Although the coronavirus might fail to treat everyone equally, it does reinforce the notion, if not the reality, that we all live in the same world. Unlike in the last recession, this time the rich and powerful cannot take their money and leave. With airports shuttered, the elites have no emergency exit; in the time of the plague, there are no distinctions between what David Goodhart described as 'people from anywhere' and 'people from somewhere'.[6] The coronavirus has placed everyone on a common ground, and this time 'people from anywhere' are desperately looking for their somewhere. But living in the same world is not the same as living in a shared world or a fair world. In normal times, the elites can afford to travel. In the time of COVID-19, they can afford to stay at home.

In the classic twentieth-century nightmare, a nuclear war threatens to kill everybody at the same time. However, in the case of the coronavirus, those young Europeans who inanely decided to party during the pandemic risked being sick for a short time, while their parents and grandparents were more likely to be killed. In this sense, the pandemic resembles climate change – it's a global disaster that affects us all differently.

If terrorism poses an asymmetric threat, the

coronavirus invokes asymmetric fears. The sociol-
ogist Bruno Latour has a persuasive explanation of
why nativist politicians like Donald Trump deny the
existential threat of climate change. It is not that they
are blind to the problem or that they don't trust science; what worries them is the claim that we will
either all survive or all die, while their basic political
intuition is zero-sum: for some people to survive,
others should die. They reject liberal international-
ism because it promises that global cooperation can
save us all.[7] We see a similar logic in their response to
COVID-19. Just as climate change will affect places
and people differently because of their geography,
COVID-19 also discriminates when it comes to 'pre-
existing conditions', such as being black or poor in
the US.

The coronavirus also discriminates by age in terms
of who survives infection and, as a result, has a strong
impact on intergenerational dynamics. In debates
about the risks of climate change, the young have
been critical of their parents' generation for not taking the future seriously. The coronavirus reverses
this dynamic: older members of society are more vul-
nerable and feel threatened by the unwillingness of
the young to change their way of life. If the crisis
were to last a long time, this intergenerational con-
flict would intensify. At the same time, social
distancing helps us to imagine how our parents and
grandparents are living – 'staying at home' is exactly

how they lived prior to the pandemic. Talking to my mother, I came to realize that even before the pandemic she was spending most of her time at home, fearing death, praying that her doctors were equipped to do their jobs and, like all grandmothers, waiting for her grandchildren to call.

Although COVID-19 is far more dangerous when old people get infected, it's the younger generation that will be most affected by the economic effects of the pandemic. An astonishing recent report from the US found that 52 per cent of people under the age of forty-five have either lost a job, been put on leave or had their hours reduced because of the outbreak. And it was only a decade ago that the younger generation in the West was battered by the Great Recession. Millennials in Southern Europe will now have suffered two huge crises by their mid-thirties. Forty per cent of young Italians and half of young Spanish workers did not have a job in the middle of the last decade. Researchers in the United States are beginning to talk about 'Generation C', the 'C' standing for coronavirus. This is the generation that will be shaped by this pandemic, whether they are currently newborn babies, children, students or those holding down their first job. This generation may grow up in a catastrophic recession.

COVID-19 has not simply strengthened and amplified existing social and political divides; it has also caused new ones. When governments around the world decided to apply lockdown procedures, observers were quick to notice that social distancing was for many people a middle-class luxury. Other people thought it was something else altogether – a poster that has been popular with right-wing anti-lockdown protesters in America reads 'Social Distancing = communism'. Society has also been divided between those who perform essential jobs and those who are able to work from home. The popular idea of antibody testing and issuing immunity passports is strongly favoured by the business community because it promises a more imminent opening of the economy. But it would also divide society into two distinct groups: those who could move freely and present little danger to others, and those who would be perceived as high-risk. It would be no surprise if companies were far more eager to employ those who had the antibodies.

When societies began to consider their 'exit strategy' from the lockdown, one option discussed in the UK and elsewhere was to let the young lead the way, perhaps starting by reopening schools, followed by a return to work for younger people who were less likely to become seriously ill if they became infected with coronavirus. Some policy experts suggested removing restrictions on twentysomethings who did not live with their parents, which could release some

4.2 million people. Some joked that a 'youth first' policy might result in a 'maximum age for drinking in pubs'. All these policies create winners and losers, and if COVID-19 restrictions last long enough, they will remake our societies.

3. Democracy as a Dictatorship of Comparisons

According to an April 2020 report by openDemocracy, more than two billion people then lived in countries in which parliaments had been suspended or restricted by coronavirus emergency measures.[1] But it is not just parliament. The lockdowns have also diminished the role of the courts. People are banned from leaving their homes. Elections are either suspended or are held in an atmosphere that makes fair political competition impossible. Media restrictions have proliferated; and while the pandemic has made reliable information more important than ever before, the economic crisis threatens the financial survival of media outlets.

Many political analysts fear that the pandemic will usher populists to power, and that once in charge these demagogues will use the crisis to suffocate democracy and impose a type of authoritarian rule. The long-term political consequence of COVID-19, the argument goes, will be restrictive legislation that will remain in force long after the coronavirus is defeated. Finally, they suggest, the most significant geopolitical outcome of the crisis will be the increase in China's global influence.

I share most of these fears. COVID-19 is particularly dangerous for those individuals with 'pre-existing conditions', and Western liberal democracies have in the last decade been suffering from considerable dysfunction, with trust in their democratic systems in dramatic decline. Populist parties have been on the rise in angry and frustrated societies. The titles of two influential recent books speak to this idea: *How Democracies Die*, by Steven Levitsky and Daniel Ziblatt,[2] and *How Democracy Ends*, by David Runciman.[3] It is logical to expect that COVID-19 will strengthen – and even accelerate – at least some of the negative political trends that preceded the crisis. Although such concerns about the future of democracy in Europe are valid, my sense is that the picture is more complicated but perhaps not as bleak.

Will COVID-19 Bring Populists to Power?

'Fear exceeds all other disorders in intensity,' remarked Michel de Montaigne. And fear is what brings populists to power. We should therefore not be surprised that many people believe that right-wing populists will be the biggest beneficiaries of the COVID-19 crisis. But is the rise of populism during the last decade better explained by fear or anxiety?

While psychologists suggest that fear and anxiety are close relatives – both contain the idea of danger – they also stress that fear is a reaction to a specific and observable danger, such as the fear of being infected with a deadly disease. By contrast, anxiety is a diffuse, unfocused, objectless belief about one's future. People are anxious that their children will have a life worse than their own. That migrants will replace them. They're anxious about the oncoming climate apocalypse, or about the prospect of alien invasion. Anxious people are also angry, while fearful people do not have the luxury of anger, because they are too busy working to survive.

Populists have been able to skilfully exploit the anger of the anxious. Anxious people do not behave in the same was as fearful people. A large and growing literature in social psychology argues that, under conditions of fear, 'people develop a heightened mindfulness and self-awareness about the constraints on free action, and take, as a central goal, the desire to restore a higher degree of coherence and certainty'.[4] In his memoir, the literary critic Marcel Reich-Ranicki gives us a powerful insight into the one-dimensional nature of the fearful mind: he confessed that in his months in the Warsaw Ghetto during the Second World War, although he spent all his time reading, he did not once pick up a novel, because he feared that if he started one he would die before he had finished it.

When the most acute stage of the current crisis is over and people cease fearing for their lives, anger will return, and populist politicians like Marine Le Pen or Matteo Salvini are likely to flourish once again. In the early days of the crisis, however, it is the intensity of the fear caused by COVID-19 that explains why it is government rather than populist rhetoric that has won the day. As the approval ratings of Merkel and Conte grow, the support for their populist challengers declines. Rather than looking for someone to express their frustration, fearful people look for somebody to protect them and turn to those with knowledge. As a result, COVID-19 has changed the public's attitude towards expertise. It has made explicit the social benefits of a competent government, in contrast with the mistrust of experts and technocracy that followed the financial crisis.

Why Wannabe Tyrants Abhor the Plague

In the opening scene of Sophocles' *Oedipus Rex*, the eponymous hero struggles to identify the cause of a plague laying waste to his city, Thebes. As it turns out, the outbreak was not only provoked by his own actions but can be wiped out only by his own death or banishment. Re-read today, this story suggests that 'the god of plague' can destroy any ruler who stakes his reputation on defeating it. Could this be why so many leaders obsessed with projecting an image of their own omnipotence have met the current pandemic with magical thinking, cowardly blame-shifting and a weirdly dazed immobility?

More than any other crisis, a public health emergency can induce people voluntarily to accept restrictions on their liberties in the hope of improving their personal security. Invasive surveillance systems and bans on freedom of assembly have been introduced and accepted around the world with little public push-back. And the striking example of Hungary's Viktor Orbán, who has given himself the power to rule by decree and destroy political opponents in the name of combating the virus, gives us grounds to fear that the current health crisis (and the economic downturn that it has set in motion) can embolden other populists in their quest for unchecked power. But are the restrictions on individual freedom imposed in response to COVID-19, restrictions that disallow not only anti-government protests but also strutting military parades and strident pro-government rallies, genuinely favourable to authoritarian concentrations or seizures of power?

Political theorists are right that authoritarian leaders thrive on crises and that they are fluent in the politics of fear. Yet not all crises are amenable to authoritarian solutions. Nor does every form of public fear accrue to the benefit of political power. The crises that authoritarians most enjoy are those that they have manufactured themselves, or that at least permit them to showcase their imagined strengths.

Carl Schmitt said that dictators aspire to wield the power of God to work miracles. But the Almighty is never asked to solve problems thrust upon Him by an unpredictably changing world that He has not created and over which He exercises minimal control.

The last-minute cancellation of presidential elections in Poland, previously scheduled for 10 May 2020, is a good example of how COVID-19 can thwart populist power-grabs rather than helping populists take control. The government was determined to organize elections in the midst of the pandemic against the will of the majority of the population, assured by the opinion polls that their candidate would easily win then but might not fare so well later when the public had had a chance to evaluate the ruling party's response to the crisis. As one opposition candidate remarked, commenting on the decision to postpone the elections: 'It turns out that reality is not as flexible as Jarosław Kaczyński's mind.'

Only by displaying their unconstrained freedom to choose which crisis warrants a response can leaders project an image of godlike power. COVID-19 has eliminated this freedom to choose. In pre-COVID Russia, President Vladimir Putin could easily 'solve' one crisis by conjuring up another. He managed to reverse the decline of his popularity following the protest movement of 2011–12 by dramatically annexing Crimea. In pre-COVID America, long before he assured the public that the coronavirus would soon miraculously disappear, US President Donald Trump recklessly dismantled the federal government's emergency-response capacity on the apparent assumption that only emergencies of his own imagining, such as migrant caravans from Mexico, would occur.

As a seemingly unstoppable crisis that has riveted the attention of the global public, COVID-19 deprives authoritarian and authoritarian-minded leaders of the chance to manufacture a 'better crisis'. Far from citing the coronavirus crisis to justify an increase in power, a high-profile slew of populists and autocrats have strenuously and ridiculously denied the very existence of the pandemic. Among them we find the Brazilian president Jair Bolsonaro, the Belarusian strongman Alexander Lukashenko, Turkmenistan's autocratic president Gurbanguly Berdymukhamedov and the Nicaraguan dictator Daniel Ortega. A professor of international relations in São Paulo has labeled them the 'Ostrich Alliance'. But they are not the only aspiring tyrants who, afraid of appearing helpless in the face of a raging plague, have plunged their heads into the sands of COVID denialism.

Political leaders in general prefer 'enemies' who can unconditionally surrender to anonymous 'threats' that need to be managed over time. Would-be dictators, in particular, find it more rewarding to pose as 'deciders' than to do the hard work required of 'problem-solvers'. The former allows them to vaunt their I-alone-can-solve-it unilateralism, while the latter requires them to cooperate with others, to freely admit their own mistakes, and to spend the time needed to master complex and evolving situations. Flashy stunts by men-of-action must give way to slow and laborious efforts by anonymous professionals. It is not only that authoritarian leaders despise crises that they do not freely choose and which require them to stake their prestige on cooperatively resolving problems that, at the outset, are difficult to understand; they also spurn 'exceptional situations' that compel them to respond with standardized rules and protocols rather than with ad hoc, discretionary moves. Mundane behaviours such as social distancing, self-isolation and washing hands are the best way to stop the spread of the disease. The leader's strokes of genius, inviting thunderous applause, are perfectly irrelevant. Worse still, the palpable courage of ICU doctors and nurses makes phony heroics in presidential palaces appear even more pathologically narcissistic than before.

Unlike democratic leaders, who can suffer defeat on a policy initiative and still manage to govern, authoritarian leaders follow the maxim: 'never show weakness'. This is yet another reason why COVID-19, which gives no signs of abating anytime soon, has proved particularly unwelcome to rulers obsessed with projecting an image of indomitable power. That the virus is indifferent to governmental edicts is obvious. Even worse for the optics of authority, citizen compliance with phase-two government orders to restart the economy is likely to be much less deferential than citizen compliance with instructions to keep their families safe.

COVID-19 also compels leaders to share both power and the political limelight with epidemiologists and other experts. In the COVID-19 world, a political leader risks losing all credibility if he continues to reward personal loyalty over technical competence, dismisses mask-wearing as an expression of political correctness or pontificates from the stage without being accompanied by medical specialists. Up-to-date information and professional advice are what matter to a frightened public. More rhetorically hyped xenophobia and political polarization have marginal appeal at best. This must be especially grating to leaders who have risen to power by dismissing all discomfiting information as political and ideological. Contrary to their basic instincts, many would-be authoritarians are being forced by the pandemic into a system of power-sharing and even podium-sharing that they may inwardly despise but cannot politically avoid.

A final feature of the current pandemic that causes problems for aspiring authoritarians is the global nature of the crisis. The ubiquity of the disease makes it possible for people to compare the actions of their own governments with the actions of other governments around the world. Success or failure at flattening the curve provides a common metric, making cross-national comparisons possible and putting strong pressure on governments that had previously succeeded in insulating themselves from public criticism. The opening provided by easy government-to-government comparisons gives citizens a capacity to grade their government's performance. This is a problem for authoritarian regimes and authoritarian-minded leaders, who previously got away with staged 'performances' supplemented by the silencing of whistle-blowers and critics.

We are just at the beginning of what promises to be a long-term crisis. It is therefore too soon to make any definitive judgement about which governments have dealt most effectively with the unfolding pandemic and its radiating consequences. But we can already see how some of the world's most prominent populists and authoritarians are being swept to ruin by the god of plague, just as Sophocles would have led us to expect.

Will the Coronavirus Benefit the 'Chinese Model'?

Like many others, in the early days of the crisis I had the impression that China would be the country that emerged from the pandemic on the strongest strategic footing. The crisis seems to have legitimized authoritarian states to those people that live in them, and early data shows that the pandemic has made Chinese citizens more critical of the American model.[5] The fact that China was the first country to be struck by the virus meant that it was also the first to start its economic recovery, which worked in its favour.

However, I'm now less certain that China will be the major beneficiary of the crisis. Anti-Chinese sentiment has increased following the revelation that the Chinese government lied to the world about the numbers of people who had died of coronavirus and were infected with it. Beijing's aggressive public relations campaign aiming to portray China as the model for effective response to the pandemic and the only global-minded power at the point when the virus was spreading to Europe and other parts of the world backfired. German public opinion was outraged to learn that Chinese diplomats had pressed German officials to praise publicly the Chinese response to the crisis.[6] Furthermore, China is likely to be negatively affected by the 'de-globalization' that will be a social and economic consequence of the pandemic. In the first quarter of 2020, China experienced its first major GDP decline since Mao's Cultural Revolution, posing a significant and symbolic challenge to a regime whose legitimacy relies on its capacity to deliver increasing living standards. It could turn out that Chinese leader Xi Jinping will be much weakened by this crisis.

Our current moment is somewhat akin to the crisis of the 1970s, when Soviet communism and Western democracies were both riven by internal turmoil during what the political philosopher Pierre Hassner called a period of 'competitive decadence'. Instead of answering the question of whether liberal democracy or Chinese-style authoritarianism is the type of regime best suited to the demands of the twenty-first century, COVID-19 achieved something else: it ended the possibility of Chinese–American cooperation in managing the problems of globalization and further eroded trust in multilateral institutions like the World Health Organization. The trend of global fragmentation and regionalization has only been strengthened. Wang Jisi, a professor at Peking University, correctly claims that the fallout from the virus has left China–US relations at their worst point since formal ties were established in the 1970s, with bilateral economic and technological decoupling 'already irreversible'.[7]

The rivalry between China and America will not trigger the return of a Cold War. Unlike the Soviet regime, the Chinese model is not an ideological alternative to capitalism but rather a part of global capitalism. However, a confrontation between the two powers will very much feel like a Cold War. As John Updike's character Harry 'Rabbit' Angstrom remarked, 'Without the Cold War, what's the point of being an American?'[8] It is clear that, regardless of the outcome of the American presidential elections in November 2020, Washington's position towards Beijing will toughen. Chinese leaders would also probably agree that without a Cold War there would be little point in continuing to incorrectly call themselves communists. Mobilizing anti-Western nationalism would be the Communist Party's best strategy to preserve its power.

When the Crowd Vanishes

Italo Calvino's novel *The Watcher*[9] tells the story of an election suffused with madness, passion and reason. The protagonist, Amerigo Ormea, a leftist intellectual, agrees to be an election monitor in Turin's Cottolengo Hospital for Incurables, a home for the mentally ill and disabled. Ever since voting became compulsory in Italy after the Second World War, such places have been particular targets of recruitment for right-wing Christian Democrats. During the election, newspapers are filled with stories about invalids and the elderly, paralysed by arteriosclerosis, being pressured to vote conservative.

Despite this, it is in Cottolengo that Ormea falls under democracy's spell. He is mesmerized by how the ritual of elections triumphs over the march of the fascists and how they give meaning to human life. What he finds most striking is the egalitarianism of democracy; the fact that all people, whether rich or poor, educated or illiterate, each have one vote of equal value. Elections resemble death, since they force you to look backwards and forwards, to both evaluate your life and to imagine another. It is in the Hospital for the Incurables that Ormea appreciates democracy's genius to turn madness into reason and passions into interests.

It is democracy's talent to misrepresent that makes Amerigo Ormea a believer, and it is its mystique rather than its transparency that converts him. Elections give every citizen a voice, but under the condition that they will not represent the intensity of their beliefs. It is this mystique of democracy that is under threat, in a world in which social distancing has been internalized as responsible behaviour. Would Amerigo Ormea have been so converted by democracy if people were only able to vote by post? It is the possibility that COVID-19 will keep us off the streets for several years rather than for several months that is the gravest danger for European liberal democracies. If we trust Bill Gates, we should expect that in the coming years 'people can get out, but not as often, and not to crowded places. Picture restaurants that only seat people at every other table, and airplanes where every middle seat is empty.'[10]

In a democracy, citizens need to be able to vote, politicians need to be able to deliberate, and people need to be able to move about, meet and act collectively.

It is also of critical importance that people have the possibility to be part of a crowd, a collective body that can express the intensity of their political passion; electoral rallies and mass demonstrations give citizens a sense of belonging that participation in elections fails to provide.

Twentieth-century democratic politics were animated by the power of the crowd. 'No one could avoid encountering them on streets and squares,' wrote Siegfried Kracauer, recalling the situation after the First World War. 'These masses were more than a weighty social factor, they were as tangible as any individual.'[11] Some theorists of democracy feared the masses, because of their 'insanity' and the danger that they could be mobilized by autocratic leaders, but they were also aware of the importance of street politics for the proper functioning of democracy. It is the possibility that crowds can reflect the intensity of political passions that reconciles many political activists with democracy. Reflecting on his participation in the famous 15 July 1927 mass political demonstration by Social Democrats in Vienna, Elias Canetti wrote, 'It was the closest thing to a revolution that I have physically experienced. Since then, I have known quite precisely that I would not have to read a single word about the storming of the Bastille. '[12]

If in the twentieth century the future of democracy was threatened by the power of crowds, now it is threatened by the prospect of the disappearance of crowds. In the last decade, those whom Thomas Friedman calls 'the square people'[13] have been a constant presence in global politics. More than ninety countries around the world have witnessed major mass protests. Millions of people have turned out to mount sizeable and sustained actions that bypass political parties, distrust the mainstream media, have few specific leaders and mostly leave formal organization aside. The *gilets jaunes* in France and Extinction Rebellion are two faces of this diverse phenomenon. Online activism is often unable to inject the sense of meaning and belonging that is the distinctive feature of street politics, and instead often resorts to cheap 'clicktivism'.

COVID-19 threatens this essential element of democratic politics; democracy cannot function if people have to stay indoors. As the technology analyst Benedict Evans recently observed, 'We are all online now, and, just as importantly, we're all willing to use this for any part of our lives, if you can work out the right experience and business model. Today, anyone will do anything online.'[14] He may be right, but it is my conviction that democracy cannot survive in the absence of 'square people' and, no less important, that the disappearance of these people may in the eyes of many indicate the end of democracy. It is impossible for me to imagine that democracies will be able to survive if we cannot gather in groups of more than fifty people. The loss of angry crowds who can freely express their discontent and demands on the streets of Western capitals blurs the distinction between liberal democracy and its poisonous doubles. In an age in which many authoritarian regimes use managed elections as a way of justifying their power, it is the freedom of citizens to go on the streets and protest and after that safely return home that is the most visible difference between free and unfree societies.

Empowered by Comparing

Doing as others do can save your life. In 2015, Al-Shabaab militants stormed the Garissa University College in Kenya and took students hostage, showing mercy only to those who could prove they were Muslims by reciting a tract from the Koran. Those who could not were shot on the spot. One Christian student saw what was happening to those in front of her and hurriedly memorized the tract. As Michelle Baddeley argues in *Copycats and Contrarians*, the girl 'saved her own life through social learning, by gathering information about others' choices and their consequences'.[15]

Such copycat logic explains the central paradox of the global response to the coronavirus outbreak. The crisis has forced societies to retreat to a 'stay-at-home nationalism' rather than a more familiar mode of cooperation. Despite this, governments have been enthusiastic to each use a similar package of policies designed to halt the transmission of the virus, despite the fact that social traditions, political regimes and public health systems vary significantly from state to state.

Why have governments that are vastly different adopted the same policy approaches? The answer might lie in the distinction between the 'politics of uncertainty' and the 'politics of risk' that the economist Frank Knight established in his landmark 1921 work, *Risk, Uncertainty and Profit*.[16] Knight claimed that, while the future is unknowable, risk is measurable, and past events can be assessed using empirical data. Uncertainty, on the other hand, applies to outcomes that we cannot predict or that we are unable to predict.

The COVID-19 pandemic has been one such moment of uncertainty. In the early stages of the crisis, when mass testing was impossible, governments were not able to weigh the costs and benefits of social distancing policies or economic shutdowns – the most responsible course of action was to assume the worst and adopt the most risk-averse position. Governments are used to managing risk, but dealing with uncertainty is a very different game.

In uncertain situations, governments must be ready to take extraordinary measures, even when they are not confident of the outcomes. At the same time, they want to avoid taking any course of action that could later be questioned by citizens familiar with what was being implemented elsewhere. Doing as others do becomes critically important in reassuring the public that the situation is under control – in the case of the coronavirus pandemic, that meant persuading them of the necessity of staying at home, wearing masks, closing businesses and complying with whatever additional policies were put in place.

Imagine that half the countries in the world had decided to proceed with a lockdown, while the others on the example of Sweden had chosen to avoid strict measures; the political pressure on both sides to change course would have been almost unbearable. Had some democratic governments introduced a state of emergency and others not done so, despite the figures for people infected of and dying from the virus being comparable, such diverse responses might have provoked a collapse in public confidence. It is easy to see why governments chose to copy the policies adopted by the countries that were hit earliest by the pandemic, even if they were unconvinced that they represented the best approach.

In this sense, copycat government policies are fundamentally different from the behaviour of the Kenyan Christian girl. Governments copy others not because they saw their policies succeeding – but because they had no idea of what would work.

Although the adoption of similar policies has helped governments to evade responsibility, over time they have increasingly been compared. Comparisons are a constant feature of any politics, but citizens usually measure the performance of a government in contrast with the efficiency of previous governments or with the promises of the opposition. COVID-19 has established a different type of comparison, with citizens comparing their government's performance with those in other countries in real time. The public are eager to know why Germany is testing more aggressively than France, why more people are dying in the UK than in Austria, and why some governments are prepared to spend much more than others in compensating people and businesses for the cost of the crisis. COVID-19 has transformed political debate, in the sense that the response of governments to the public health and economic challenges presented by the pandemic is the only thing that matters. It has created the illusion that the performance of a government can be objectively measured, and it is this comparison rather than criticism of the opposition that shapes governments' decisions most. For instance, it is the fact that Austria has decided to loosen restrictions that is responsible for the cracks in political consensus that have appeared in Germany.

That most governments decided to impose lockdown and introduce emergency legislation explains why people all over the world were ready to accept the violation of their privacy in the fight against COVID-19. But the hegemony of their approach also means that, as some governments decide to suspend the restrictions, those who decide to prolong them are exposed. The paradox of this crisis is that it has given governments extraordinary powers, while also empowering every citizen by allowing them to judge whether their government is doing better or worse than others.

During the pandemic, the success of any government's policies has been dependent on the active support of its citizens. Any individual who decides to violate the politics of social distancing is an obstacle to the government's objectives; in this sense, a state of emergency restricts citizens' rights but paradoxically increases their power.

But empowerment by comparison ends when countries start exiting from the lockdown and when economic concerns replace public health concerns. Should we be more interested in the number of the newly infected or the number of unemployed, or what the state is doing to support businesses?

This is when citizens who in the early stage of the pandemic were empowered by comparing the performance of their government with that of other governments can end up disoriented and disempowered. This is when fear gives way to anger as the prevailing mood in a society.

Turning Schmitt on His Head

In the late eighteenth century, Jeremy Bentham designed an institutional form that he called 'the panopticon'. The concept behind it was to allow a watchman to observe all the inmates in an institution – whether a prison, school or hospital – without them knowing whether they were being watched. The design soon became a symbol of our modern understanding of the use of power to control dangerous individuals or groups. The nineteenth-century politician and anarchist Pierre-Joseph Proudhon famously declared that 'to be governed is to be watched over, inspected, spied on, directed, legislated at, regulated, docketed, indoctrinated, preached at, controlled, assessed, weighed, censored and ordered about.'[17] Many will agree that little has changed since Proudhon's days, other than technology.

In moments of crisis, the idea of the panopticon frequently rears its head. The emergence of the state-imposed public health surveillance that many fear will be the unintended outcome of the COVID-19 pandemic might be regarded as the newest incarnation of Bentham's project. The difference is that, while the original panopticon asked people to strip naked for the government in exchange for protection against dangerous elements, in our latter-day version the state promises to use public health surveillance to protect people from themselves.

On 26 February 2020, when the scale of the pandemic in his country was still unclear, the Italian philosopher Giorgio Agamben wrote a controversial op-ed claiming that the emergency measures introduced by the Italian government were entirely disproportionate. 'What is once again manifested is the tendency,' Agamben asserted, 'to use a state of exception as a normal paradigm of government.'[18] He shared a view that the government's response to COVID-19 was a manifestation of 'the tyrannical instinct' of liberal governments and an opportunity to bring back emergency measures that were reminiscent of those used during the 'war on terror'. Just as those people who were troubled by the shutting of European borders tended to perceive COVID-19 as the return of the refugee crisis, many human rights practitioners fear that, when the virus is defeated, the surveillance practices will live on. To them, a 'state of exception' is nothing less than a nail in the coffin of democracy.

Are the critics of 'the state of exception' justified in interpreting the surveillance triggered by COVID-19 as the return of the West's discredited 'war on terror'? Is the 'normalization' of the violation of privacy in a pandemic as destructive to democracy as the legalization of torture advocated by George

W. Bush's government in the years following the 9/11 terror attacks?

Governments are partially to blame for the zeal of their critics, and the use of militaristic rhetoric makes it easy to see the restriction of rights as reminiscent of the post-9/11 period. But in making the fight against the virus indistinguishable from the fight against the terrorist, both of them 'invisible enemies', liberals risk falling into the 'libertarian trap'. Individual liberties are never an absolute value and should always be weighed in relation to the public good. Critics of Bush's 'war on terror' were right to insist that the state should never legalize torture; it destroys a person's dignity and was also shown not to work – it can result in false confessions. As some critics of Bush's policies argued, if government officials were compelled to torture, as in the infamous 'ticking time bomb scenario',* they should do it only as an act of civil disobedience.

However, anti-terrorist surveillance and virus-tracking apps are not the same thing. Practice shows that contact tracing helps governments contain the spread of the disease, and also that it helps medical authorities to study the disease and shorten the time

* Suppose that a person with a knowledge of an imminent terrorist attack, which will kill many people, is in the hands of the authorities and that he will disclose the information needed to prevent the attack only if he is tortured. Should he be tortured?

that it might take to find a vaccine. The surveillance used by the government in the fight against COVID-19 is no secret – people know that the government will track their contacts. And if I refuse to allow the government to track my contacts, I might be indirectly responsible for the death of another human being.

In short, the liberal defence of rights in the context of the 'war on terror' does not apply directly during this pandemic. It is not only the tendency of democratic governments to over-react in the face of a pandemic; it could be the temptation of some governments to seek to minimize the threat of the coronavirus for economic reasons that could be lethal for democracy. Should we admire the human rights activists who are suing governments for forcing people to wear masks, using anti-burqa legislation in their legal argument? Or should we rather encourage them to sue governments for forcing people to wear masks while not providing enough of them?

In his eye-opening book *Fear Itself*,[19] Ira Katznelson argued that Franklin Roosevelt succeeded in saving liberal democracy in America not by resisting extraordinary measures but rather by demonstrating the effectiveness of democracy in a time of uncertainty and fear. His strategy was to counter Carl Schmitt and demonstrate that liberal democracies, 'with their fractious parties, parliaments and polarization, could invent solutions and find their way while holding on to their core convictions and practices'.

What, in Katznelson's view, distinguishes democracy from dictatorship is not that democracy opposes the imposition of 'the state of exception', but that it does it in order to protect itself rather than because it can get away with it. However, in order for democracy to take exceptional measures while remaining true to its liberal nature, it must distinguish between temporary actions and permanent policy. Democratic actors should require that key legislative acts be temporary and subject to formal renewal. It is this principle that Viktor Orbán has decided to violate in a blunt, ham-fisted way.

Secondly, neither individual leaders nor institutions should be exempt from criticism, and policies of exception must not result in invisibility or isolation from democratic practices. To the contrary, each branch of government – the judiciary, the legislature and the executive itself – must have opportunities to share information and pass judgements in real time. Governments may bypass parliament where they have to, but they should never retire it.

Finally, opportunities for retrospective appraisal should be preserved. A process of evaluation, tied to sanctions when liberal norms have been violated, is particularly valuable for political regimes that are committed to democratic deliberation and collective choice.[20]

Which Way?

In trying to guess the direction of change, many other commentators have become preoccupied with whether democracies or authoritarian regimes deal better with the pandemic, even though it is clear that the nature of the political regime is not the critical factor explaining success or failure in containing the pandemic. As Rachel Kleinfeld has argued, 'Despite attempts by politicians to use the crisis to tout their favored political model, the record so far does not show a strong correlation between efficacy and regime type.'[21] While some autocracies, such as China and Singapore, have initially performed well, others like Iran have done very poorly. Similarly, some democracies, for example Italy and the United States, have stumbled, while others, including South Korea, Germany and Taiwan, have performed admirably. In Kleinfeld's analysis, the main factors that determine a nation's success at containing the COVID-19 pandemic are governments' previous experiences of dealing with similar crises, the level of social trust in a society, and the capacity of the state. In her view, Taiwan, South Korea, Hong Kong and Singapore, though politically diverse, learned the right lessons from the SARS epidemic in 2002–3 and developed speedy tests soon after the coronavirus began spreading, in order to try to get ahead of the virus. All of them had emergency laws that permitted the extraordinary right to track where infected individuals had been, and they relaxed privacy regulations to spread that information widely and alert people that they had been exposed to the virus and should be tested. Finally, they relied on heavily enforced quarantines to slow the spread of the outbreak.

All the countries that effectively beat back COVID-19 have high levels of public trust in their institutions; the success of governmental social control depends more on voluntary compliance than on enforcement. Although China, Singapore and South Korea have quite different political regimes, all three are in the top ten countries in the world when it comes to public trust in government. And only governments that are trusted by their citizens can effectively maintain an onerous lockdown.

Conversely, in authoritarian Iran and democratic Italy, the public's low trust in their institutions has made the introduction of social distancing more problematic. Political polarization and low trust, according to Kleinfeld, also at least partially explain the difficulties the United States has had in dealing with the crisis.

A government's capacity – its ability to intervene successfully in areas ranging from communication and health provision to quarantine maintenance and equipment manufacturing – is the third critical factor that Kleinfeld thinks has determined a successful response to the crisis. This capacity is only loosely related to a country's GDP or the character of its political regime. It is the quality of the bureaucracy that is decisive, rather than the size of the budget or even the amount of health spending.

Kleinfeld's research demonstrates that, while the coronavirus pandemic intensified the competitive propaganda between democratic and authoritarian systems, the global response to the coronavirus blurred the borders between different types of regimes. Democratic regimes were just as willing to violate the privacy of their citizens as authoritarian ones. At the same time, it was clear that authoritarian rulers were just as interested in the responses of the public as democratic politicians who fear the next election. In the words of political philosopher David Runciman, 'Under a lockdown, democracies reveal what they have in common with other political regimes: here too politics is ultimately about power and order.' In the days of the COVID-19 lockdown, all institutions and all public functions were divided between essential and non-essential ones, between those that you could send home and those whom you could not afford to send home. Unfortunately, in this divide parliaments ended on the non-essential side, and one of the legacies of the COVID-19 crisis will be a further decline of the role of parliaments at the expense of the executive power. The proliferation of contested elections could be one more outcome of the crisis. It is yet to be seen whether democracies or authoritarian regimes will be more effective in a second wave of the pandemic, but it is the internal transformation of both democratic and authoritarian regimes, rather than transition to democracy or tyranny, that will be the real political legacy of COVID-19.

In other words, the change that COVID-19 brings is not a new version – either authoritarian or democratic – of 'the end of history'; what it may bring is a less ideological but a more unstable world.

4. Are You Here?

Sometime in March 2020, during the second week of my COVID-19 confinement, a friend emailed me an amusing Venn diagram. It depicted twelve overlapping circles, each representing a popular dystopia. All the famous ones were there: *1984*, *Brave New World*, *The Handmaid's Tale*, *A Clockwork Orange* and *Lord of the Flies*. And then, it said, 'You are here', in that small area where they all intersected. Are we there indeed – living through all these nightmares simultaneously?

A century ago, the Spanish flu arrived in a world that had been torn apart, exhausted and demoralized by the Great War. It also killed like a war, with healthy adults between the ages of twenty and forty most likely to die. The epidemic was a global event, but people did not remember it as one, because the idea of a common world had collapsed during the long years of war. The COVID-19 pandemic promises to put an end to globalization as we know it. We can only speculate about whether it will occasion what is normally accomplished by wars, but, irrespective of what happens next, we can be confident that, when the virus is defeated, the world will be swept by a 'pandemic of nostalgia'.

In the seventeenth century, nostalgia was thought to be a curable but contagious malady. Its primary symptom was melancholia, which was thought to derive from a yearning either to return to one's land or for a different time. Those afflicted often complained of hearing voices and seeing ghosts. Sufferers acquired '"a lifeless and haggard countenance" and an "indifference towards everything", confusing past and present, real and imaginary events'.[1] When the pandemic is over, people will be nostalgic for that bygone era when we could easily fly to almost anywhere in the world; when restaurants were packed; and when death was so unnatural that, on an elderly person's passing away, we wondered whether their death had been caused by a doctor's mistake. But while we will be eager to return to normality, we will discover that it will be impossible to do so. There is also something disturbing about the world of yesterday. We can never know the future of the present, but we have already lived the future of the past.

During the acute phase of the crisis, we saw that national self-reliance trumps mutual interest. When Italy asked allies for urgent medical supplies, not a single EU country responded. Germany initially banned the export of medical masks and other protective gear, while France requisitioned all the face masks that it produced. The European Commission was forced to step in and regulate the export of medical equipment.

But while the return of the nation state was the inevitable response to such a massive public health danger, in a world lacking American leadership and sundered by US–China rivalry, a more united Europe and Brussels endowed with emergency powers may turn out to be the only realistic solution for dealing with the next phase of the crisis.

While the virus brought back the ghosts of the three recent crises that have shattered Europe in the last decade – the war on terror, the refugee crisis and the global financial crisis – it also shed new light on the fallout from those crises. The outcome of the global financial crisis was the unwillingness to mutualize debts and a reluctance to loosen constraints on governments' spending as a way to overcome the crisis. Now we see the opposite happening. The currently debated Recovery Fund was unthinkable a decade ago.

The European experience of the war on terror was that, unlike Americans after 9/11, Europeans were unwilling to trade their right to privacy for more security. This crisis revisits that decision. The polls indicate that the majority of people were ready to empower their governments and tolerate some violation of their right of privacy for the purpose of containing the spread of the coronavirus.

The refugee crisis ended up with the unspoken consensus that closing internal European borders was impossible and that closing the external borders of the EU is undesirable. It was common sense that, if the borders between the EU member states for one reason or the other were closed, the biggest losers would be the East Europeans. This crisis demonstrates that borders can be closed, at least for a while, and that Western Europe is then also a big loser. The organization of charter flights at the peak of the pandemic to transport seasonal workers from Eastern Europe to France, Germany and United Kingdom has dramatically changed the nature of the debate. The crisis also persuaded the majority of Europeans of the critical importance of the protection of the Union's external borders.

When Italians and Spaniards were dying by the thousand every day, Brussels had little to say. The European Union has proven structurally unsuited to ameliorating the unfolding catastrophe, an irrelevant actor at the very moment that people were seeking protection. Imprisoned in their homes, Europeans suddenly ceased thinking about the European Union. While Italians and Spaniards felt betrayed by the EU, their betrayal was focused on their fellow Europeans and their governments rather than on the European bureaucracy. When people became absorbed in trying to understand why fewer people were getting infected and dying in some European countries than in others, the idea of a common Europe disappeared. Nobody cared to count the number of dead or infected on a continental level. No government called out for European health policies or for the Euro-peanization of COVID-19-related personal data. There were times during this crisis that the European Union started to resemble the final decades of the Holy Roman Empire, when people living in the territory of the empire became unaware that they were even still a part of it. In many places in Europe, the crisis diminished citizens' interest in the EU, but at the same time it forced governments to realize their dependence on it. The COVID-19 crisis was at the same time a failure of the European Union but also a cry for more European cooperation. In the days of the quarantine, the old continent experienced its hundred days of solitude. Many in Europe have turned against China. The illusion of US–China cooperation in defence of multilateralism was over, while the image of the United States simply collapsed. This time it was not only about President Trump and his destructive policies. The majority of Europeans probably for the first time saw the US not as a global hegemon but as a broken society nobody can rely on.

The political challenge presented by COVID-19 confronted European leaders with a strategic choice: they could either fight to preserve a globalized world of open borders, or they could work towards a softer version of de-globalization. At the end of the day, they'll end up doing both. Brussels will remain the last man standing in defence of globalization, while at the same time it will try to use the pressures coming from the process of de-globalization to obtain more powers and to advocate more integration in certain areas. The globalized nature of COVID-19, combined with the realization that nineteenth-century economic nationalism is no longer an option for small and mid-sized European nation states, may give rise to a newly configured, EU-centred territorial nationalism. The coronavirus has taught Europeans that, if they want to remain safe, they cannot tolerate a world in which most medicines or masks are produced outside of Europe. Likewise, they can't rely on Chinese firms to build a European 5G network or on the United States to protect Europeans' way of life. If the world is going protectionist, effective protectionism in Europe is possible only on continental level.

The great paradox of COVID-19 is that it was the failure rather than the success of the European Union to demonstrate its relevance that urged European governments to opt for deeper integration. In a similar way, social distancing has brought the opening of the European mind. Closing the borders between EU member states and locking people in their apartments has made us more cosmopolitan than ever. For those with access to communications technology, the pandemic has not de-globalized but de-localized: our geographical neighbours are no closer than friends and colleagues abroad. And those who stay at home feel closer to the TV announcers than to their neighbours. For perhaps the first time in history, people around the world are having the same conversations and sharing the same fears. By staying at home and spending countless hours in front of computers and TV screens, people are comparing what is happening to them with what is happening to others elsewhere. It might only be for this weird moment in our history, but we cannot deny that we are currently experiencing what it feels like to live in One World.

It is one of the great optical illusions of twenty-first-century globalization that only mobile people are truly cosmopolitan and that only those who feel at home in different places can maintain a universalist perspective. And yet the ultimate cosmopolitan, Immanuel Kant, never left his hometown of Königsberg. His town at various times belonged to different empires, but he always preferred to remain there. Today's paradoxes of globalization (or de-globalization) perhaps began with him. Covid-19 has infected the world with cosmopolitanism, while turning states against globalization.

Notes

The Return of the Unresolved

1 José Saramago, *Blindness* (Harvest Books, 1999).
2 Ibid., p. 292.
3 Albert Camus, *The Plague* (New York, Vintage, 1991), p. 71.
4 Ibid., p. 183.
5 Laura Spinney, *Pale Rider: The Spanish Flu of 1918 and How It Changed the World* (London, Random House, 2017).
6 Ibid.
7 Carlo Rovelli, 'Coronavirus, a lezione di umiltà: siamo fragili ne usciremo uniti', *Corriere della Sera*, 1 April 2020: https://www.corriere.it/esteri/20_aprile_01/corona virus-lezione-umilta-siamo-fragili-ne-usciremo-uniti-6a285592-7448-11ea-b181-d5820c4838fa.shtml
8 Ibid.
9 Ivan Krastev, 'Seven Early Lessons from the Coronavirus', *European Council on Foreign Relations*, 18 March 2020: https://www.ecfr.eu/article/commentary_seven_early_lessons_from_the_coronavirus
10 Astra Taylor, 'The Rules We've Lived by Won't All Apply', in 'Coronavirus Will Change the World Permanently. Here's How', *Politico*, 19 March 2020:

https://www.politico.com/news/magazine/2020/03/19/
coronavirus-effect-economy-life-society-analysis-
covid-135579

11 Viktor Shklovsky, *Viktor Shklovsky: A Reader*, ed. Alex-
andra Berlina (Bloomsbury Academic, 2016).

12 Walter Bagehot, *The English Constitution*, ed. Paul Smith
(Cambridge University Press, 2001), p. 34.

13 Adam Tooze, 'The Normal Economy is Never Coming Back', *Foreign Policy*, 9 April 2020: https://foreign
policy.com/2020/04/09/unemployment-coronavirus-
pandemic-normal-economy-is-never-coming-back/

Stay-at-Home Nationalism

1 Chiara Pagano, 'From National Threat to Oblivion',
Eurozine, 2 April 2020: https://www.eurozine.com/
from-national-threat-to-oblivion/

2 Zygmunt Bauman, *Globalization: The Human Consequences* (Polity Press, 1998).

3 Quoted in A. Wess Mitchell and Charles Ingrao,
'Emperor Joseph's Solution to Coronavirus', *Wall
Street Journal*, 6 April 2020: https://www.wsj.com/arti
cles/emperor-josephs-solution-to-coronavirus-11586
214561

4 'Portugal to Treat Migrants as Residents during Coronavirus Crisis', *Reuters*, 28 March 2020: https://uk.
reuters.com/article/uk-health-coronavirus-portugal/
portugal-to-treat-migrants-as-residents-during-corona

virus-crisis-idUKKBN21F0MC?fbclid=IwARoacRUK
h5JwK6P0ZJo7HZeLXSR-DEWLLtog88uBj5UPAQV
vxE6rIGKhy1Y

5 Stephen Holmes, personal conversation.
6 David Goodhart, *Road to Somewhere* (Hurst & Co., 2017).
7 Bruno Latour, *Down to Earth* (Polity, 2018).

Democracy as a Dictatorship of Comparisons

1 'Alarm as 2 Billion People Have Parliaments Shut or
   Limited by COVID-19', *openDemocracy*, 8 April 2020:
   https://www.opendemocracy.net/en/5050/alarm-
   two-billion-people-have-parliaments-suspended-or-
   limited-covid-19/
2 Steven Levitsky and Daniel Ziblatt, *How Democracies
   Die* (Crown, 2018).
3 David Runciman, *How Democracy Ends* (Profile Books,
   2018).
4 Ira Katznelson, *Fear Itself: The New Deal and the Origins
   of Our Time* (Liveright, 2014), p. 33.
5 Mark Hannah and Caroline Gray, 'Global Views of
   American Democracy: Implications for Coronavirus
   and Beyond', EGF Report, April 2020: https://
   egfound.org/stories/independent-america/
   modeling-democracy/#china
6 'Germany Says China Sought to Encourage Positive
   COVID-19 Comments', *Reuters*, 26 April 2020: https://
   www.reuters.com/article/us-health-coronavirus-

germany-china/germany-says-china-sought-to-encourage-positive-covid-19-comments-idUSKCN 2280JW

7 Jamil Anderlini, 'Why China is Losing the Coronavirus Narrative', *Financial Times*, 19 April 2020: https://www.ft.com/content/8d7842fa-8082-11ea-82f6-150830 b3b99a

8 John Updike, *Rabbit at Rest* (Penguin, 1991), pp. 442–3.

9 Italo Calvino, *The Watcher and Other Stories* (Harvest, 1975).

10 'Bill Gates' Brutal Reality Check on the Coronavirus Reopening', *Axios*, 24 April 2020: https://www.axios.com/bill-gates-coronavirus-reopening-warning-a3e 14558-9b71-40b4-9ca5-16edafe67dee.html

11 Siegfried Kracauer, *From Caligari to Hitler: A Psychological History of the German Film* (Princeton University Press, 2019), p. 54.

12 Elias Canetti, *The Conscience of Words* (HarperCollins, 1979).

13 Thomas L. Friedman, 'The Square People', *New York Times*, 13 May 2014: https://www.nytimes.com/2014/05/14/opinion/friedman-the-square-people-part-1.html

14 Benedict Evans, 'COVID and Forced Experiments', ben-evans.com, 13 April 2020: https://www.ben-evans.com/benedictevans/2020/4/13/covid-and-forced-experiments

15 Michelle Baddeley, *Copycats and Contrarians* (Yale University Press, 2018), p. 6.

NOTES

16 Frank H. Knight, *Risk, Uncertainty and Profit* (The Riverside Press, 1921).

17 P.-J. Proudhon, *General Idea of the Revolution in the Nineteenth Century* (University Press of the Pacific, 2004), p. 294.

18 Giorgio Agamben, 'Lo stato d'eccezione provocato da un'emergenza immotivata', *Il Manifesto*, 26 February 2020: https://ilmanifesto.it/lo-stato-deccezione-provo cato-da-unemergenza-immotivata/?fbclid=IwAR17 ciygOzmIpolNxACx8WMoRzrPpePxJMNoTns7ni69 ZfwO_QzmHYeYXVk%5C

19 Ira Katznelson, *Fear Itself: The New Deal and the Origins of Our Time* (Liveright, 2014), p. 32.

20 Ewa Atanasow and Ira Katznelson, 'Governing Exigencies: On Liberal Democracy and National Security', in *The Governance Report 2017*, Hertie School of Governance (Oxford University Press, 2017), pp. 95–110.

21 Rachel Kleinfeld, 'Do Authoritarian or Democratic Countries Handle Pandemics Better?', CEIP Commentary, 31 March 2020: https://carnegieendowment. org/2020/03/31/do-authoritarian-or-democratic-coun tries-handle-pandemics-better-pub-81404

Are You Here?

1 Svetlana Boym , *The Svetlana Boym Reader*, eds. Cristina Vatulescu et al. (Bloomsbury Publishing USA, 2018), p. 217.

Acknowledgements

I would like to thank José Ignacio Torreblanca, who interviewed me in mid-March 2020 for the ECFR website, and pushed me to start ordering my messy reflections about the crisis we were all just entering. It was due to the persuasive insistence of my German editor Maria Barankow and my literary agent Toby Mundy that I committed to laying out my thinking at book length, and I'm thankful to them for that. Toby, as well as Lenny Benardo, accompanied me through every page of the book, giving my thoughts clarity and style. Evgeny Morozov and his Syllabus were invaluable sources of ideas and information. I am extremely grateful to Casiana Ionita at Penguin Books for the insightful remarks and suggestions that helped me to re-think the structure of the book. I also cannot thank Yana Papazova enough for her support. Alex Soros, Alexander Andreev, Antoinette Primatarova, Bilyana Kourtasheva, Bruce Jackson, Clemena Antonova, Daniel Smilov, Dessi and Anri Kissilenko, Deyan Kiuranov and Lili Alexandrieva, Georgi Gospodinov, Ivan Vejvoda, Ludger Hagedorn, Mila Ganeva, Milla Mineva, Milos Vec, Momchil Metodiev, Nev Andreeva, Nick Humphrey, Ralitsa Peeva, Ruzha Smilova, Stephen Holmes, Thomas

Bagger, Venelin Ganev and Vessela Tcherneva all contributed valuable comments that helped make the book intellectually much more complex. I owe them all my gratitude, while the book's deficiencies remain entirely my own responsibility.